CW00842868

Clear Addictions to Prescriptions

Resolving Side-Effects of Pharmaceuticals While Restoring Physical & Mental Health

By Dr. Alexander Haskell, ND

Copyright © 2018 by Dr. Alexander Haskell, ND

All rights reserved.

ISBN-13: 978-1984037732
ISBN-10: 1984037730

Table of Contents

INTRODUCTION

IV NAD therapy for addictions was introduced outside the United States about 20 years ago but now, in a limited number of treatment centers across the United States, it has become the primary therapy for the recovery from addictions.

There is little doubt about the benefits of IV NAD, but it is not a panacea.

We started using IV NAD about eight years, with some responses bordering on the miraculous, while others less dramatic, and often with moderate relapses of physical and mental symptoms within a couple of months.

Over the years we realized that if other underlying health issues were not simultaneously investigated and corrected, then the benefits of NAD would only be partial.

Since we've expanded our IV NAD Program to address and correct underlying biochemical and hormonal issues, as well as improving the pathways of detoxification, we truly believe that our approach is a broad leap beyond any other treatment center, including those offering IV NAD.

NAD certainly remains our core therapy for recovery but unless it is incorporated into a broad, holistic approach.

We feel it is important for you to understand the details of our approach and how our program is tailored for each individual.

So please take your time to read each chapter in sequence, because each chapter builds upon the others.

In part, your recovery depends upon becoming educated,

upon your participation and dedication, and upon understanding the ways and means of recovering your health.

Recovery

If you've experienced rehab, very likely you know its pitfalls and false promises, and may still be questioning why it didn't work for you.

If you've been able to stop your prescription, you know your health still isn't what it should be.

You may feel frustrated because of side-effects, poor quality of life and health, and thinking there must be a way out.

You'd give anything to have your physical and mental health back again.

This book is dedicated, in part, to education, to explain how to be free of your prescription(s) and their side-effects, and, more importantly, how to recover and resurrect your physical and mental health.

I shall not place the primary blame upon the multi-national, multi-billion-dollar for-profit pharmaceutical corporations, but rather upon us, the people, who remain naïve and gullible about the underlying motivations of drug companies, ignorant about the mysterious innate intelligence we all possess, and uneducated about the prevention of disease and the maintenance of health.

Like children, we have surrendered ourselves to a system which has little to do with health and wellness, and everything to do with creating a need (addiction) for medication.

We genuflect to authority and often relinquish our intuition, common sense and inquisitive nature.

We visit our physician, hoping to know <u>what</u> we are suffering from, yet, in the end, we should be asking, "Why? What are the <u>reasons</u> I feel the way I do?"

But we naively accept our prescription, which is nothing more than a synthetic chemical and completely foreign to the human body, without asking for an explanation.

This needs to become the primary question which you, and your physician, should be asking, "Why am I not well?"

We are naïve to think that drugs will ever resolve the reasons we are unwell.

We are ignorant to think that drugs will restore our health and well-being.

In fact, drugs move us in the opposite direction, towards ill-health, for two reasons.

The first is this. Every physician knows that most drugs, if administered in too high a dose, are lethal, because they are a poison to the human body.

So, what about a small dose of poison every day?

Use your common sense.

If a large dose is lethal, because it's a poison, then a small, seemingly harmless dose will, if taken daily, veer us off the path leading to health and take us into a wasteland of side-effects.

The physical and mental changes we experience are very subtle, until one day we wake up to realize that maybe the reason we don't feel well is because of the prescription.

The second reason drugs lead us away from health is because the underlying causes, which caused your symptoms in the first place, which brought you to seek the help of your physician, have not been investigated, addressed or resolved.

They still remain even though the drug is masking their symptoms.

One Analogy of Drug Side-Effects

Here we have a bowl, which represents the vessel of the human body.

Using this analogy, environmental toxins and chemicals, including prescription drugs, are poured into this bowl, and when it becomes full and cannot hold any more, these chemical residues begin to spill over the side.

This spilling represents the time when physical and mental symptoms appear.

This is a well-known viewpoint of physicians practicing environmental medicine, that chemical toxins and their residues will cause symptoms.

It is obvious then, that the way to reduce symptoms related to drugs and toxic environmental chemicals is to stop filling the bowl, BUT the bowl remains full.

Even if we stop filling the bowl, which is impossible when living in our polluted world, we are still going to experience some degree of physical and mental symptoms.

The approach of our rehab centers is to stop filling the bowl, but for true recovery and the restoration of health, we need to empty the bowl using various detoxification and purification therapies.

It May Not Be Just Your Prescription

I wish to make two important points here.

The 1st is, your health is determined by, or a reflection of, the function of all your cells.

If the cells of your body and brain are not functioning optimally then you will experience symptoms.

So, if we want to empty the bowl to recover your health, you must be thinking on the cellular level.

If we can clear toxins and drug residues from inside your cells, then they will function optimally and your overall health and vitality will be restored.

The 2nd point is, people believe their symptoms, or side-effects, are due to their prescription, that in order to feel well again, they must simply stop their prescription.

This is totally naïve.

I will remind you again and again, your physical and mental symptoms are not solely due to your prescription, but also from chemicals and pollutants accumulated over your lifetime and two other primary causes.

THREE PRIMARY CAUSES OF PHYSICAL & MENTAL SYMPTOMS

To understand how to stop your prescription, minimize side-effects and to recover your physical and mental health, we must start at the beginning, the rudiments of health and disease.

To begin, there is no disconnect between your body and your brain.

What happens in your body affects your brain and emotions, and what happens in your brain (*thoughts, beliefs, joys, fears, etc.*) affects the functions of your body.

So let's develop a foundation, a way of understanding how and WHY we develop chronic physical and mental symptoms.

If we understand these reasons or causes, then we can not only prevent illness but reverse it.

There are three primary causes of illness.

The 1st cause is nutritional deficiencies. If your cells do not have the nutrients they require then their function declines and you will experience symptoms.

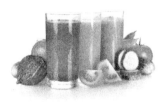

The 2nd cause is pathogens (*bacteria, viruses, mold and parasites*). You might be surprised how many people have low-grade, silent, systemic infections without even knowing it, and neither do their physicians.

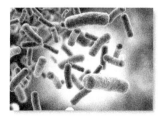

7

Pathogens excrete their toxins (*biotoxins*) which seep into our cells, adding another reason for a decline in cellular function and the onset of symptoms. These biotoxins fill our bowl.

The 3rd cause is environmental chemicals and toxins in the air we breathe, the food and water we ingest, the cosmetics we apply to our skin, and synthetic drugs.

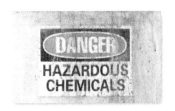

The holistic approach to recovering your physical and mental health must therefore include the following;

- **Nutritional Deficiencies:** Increase the intake of nutrient dense foods, ensure the complete digestion of food and improve the assimilation of nutrients through the small intestines into the body.
- **Pathogens:** Determine if pathogens are present and use various therapies to reduce their population while simultaneously improving immune function.
- **Toxic Residues:** Reduce exposure to toxins and use various purification therapies to empty the bowl.

I repeat, your symptoms are partly due to your prescription but also because of the three primary causes of illness.

Remember, the goal is not to just get off drugs to reduce side-effects but to restore your health and vitality by addressing the numerous causes of physical and mental ill-health.

INTRODUCTION TO MEDICINE

Our present medical system, born in the antibiotic era, has existed for a relatively brief period and that what is now labeled as alternative, has a rich history all the way back to Hippocrates.

Today, people are waking up to the fact that modern medicine, when addressing chronic ailments, has its drawbacks.

Prescriptions do not 'cure' chronic ailments. They certainly offer relief, at least temporarily, but in the end, they do nothing to restore health.

And shouldn't this be the primary goal of our healthcare system?

But people are beginning to realize, they must become involved and become an active participant if they are going to recover their health.

People want to become educated and to work in partnership with their physician.

They want to know those factors which promote or sabotage their health.

They are beginning to recognize and honor the body's innate capacity to heal, and learning how to trust and listen to their instincts, intuition and innate common sense.

Tipping the Scales

To add a second point of view around why we develop symptoms, we'll use the Libra Scale.

At birth the scale is tipped to one side, let's say all the way to the right, which represents health and vitality.

With this analogy, on the right side we place everything which promotes health, including sunlight, fresh air, clean water, nutrient dense foods, a clean shelter, love, movement, creativity and a spiritual orientation to life.

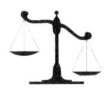

On the left side we place everything which is harmful and destructive to life, including pollution, synthetic chemicals, drugs, stress and anxiety, pathogens, a sense of isolation and many others.

With the scales tipped toward health, to the right, as we load insults onto the left, our scale begins to gradually tip towards the left.

This gradual tipping represents the onset of mild physical and mental symptoms.

Obviously, to feel better we must place more benefits on the right side and remove harmful insults from the left.

But what do most people naively do?

They turn to an over-the-counter medication or a prescription to reduce their symptoms.

In terms of the scale, these drugs would be placed on the left side. The person is feeling relief, but the scale is now tipped even more to left.

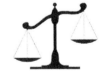

In most cases, nothing beneficial is placed on the right, nor removed from the left.

Over time, if corrections are not made, the scales will tip all the way to the left and now we have a chronic condition or pathology.

At this point, no matter how many beneficial things we load onto the right side, no matter how many supplements we take, we will never regain our health, until we also remove things from the left.

I think these two models, the bowl and Libra Scale, provide a good overview of a holistic approach to recovery.

Traditional vs. Alternative

As you can see, there's a wide gap between the approach of our present medical system and the alternative.

Taking a prescription or over-the-counter medication will do nothing to shift the Libra Scale to the right and will continue to fill the bowl.

The intention of most drugs is to reduce symptoms, but they also silence your innate wisdom's attempt to communicate to you that something is wrong, that something is out of balance.

If you become educated, if you develop a positive attitude about your present condition, if you engage and participate in your recovery, then the journey you are on will bear fruit.

Basic Naturopathic Principles

Illness does not arrive like a thief in the night but gradually and silently seeps into our lives.

I believe that under utopian conditions (environmental, social, financial & political) we should be able to live life in perfect health.

Yet this ideal will never be the case unless we are hypervigilant, inquisitive and develop a spiritual practice.

We can no longer entrust our health to a corporate run government and for-profit pharmaceutical corporations.

So where do we start?

How can each person begin to recover their health?

How do we plant our feet onto a new path that leads us towards greater vitality?

The starting point must begin with education and a new enlightened perspective.

Symptoms Are the Messenger

I strongly believe that everyone possesses the capacity to heal, and I refer to this capacity as an innate wisdom which is superior in knowledge to the most enlightened physician.

In pre-med, I was extremely fortunate to have a professor who continually reminded us of this miraculous, incomprehensible capacity which monitors, regulates and corrects any deviation from 'normal.'

I've come to understand more deeply how this wisdom untiringly maintains this balance from the moment of our conception, day in and day out, until this present moment in time.

Describing this faculty as miraculous is an understatement.

This means that each one of us has their own physician to call upon, which communicates to us through the language of physical and mental symptoms.

These symptoms can appear in an acute situation or the milder onset of chronic symptoms such as aches and pains, dizziness, fatigue, headaches or digestive issues.

These symptoms communicate to us that something is not right, that we need to investigate the underlying reasons for them rather than immediately turning to some medication for relief.

I believe this is the most important mindset for anyone trying to recover their health; there are always reasons, always causes for why we experience unpleasant symptoms.

And with this, we begin to nurture an attitude, that symptoms are the voice of our innate physician attempting to get our attention, and to bring us back into balance.

Through our attentiveness and appreciation for this wisdom within, we can then participate in assisting this intelligence during the process of recovery and regulation.

The Three Primary Causes of Chronic Illness

Let's cover, in greater detail, the primary underlying causes of physical and mental symptoms.

Nutritional Deficiencies

Over 2,000 years ago the Father of Medicine, Hippocrates, believed chronic ailments had two primary causes.

The 1st cause was nutritional deficiencies.

This is simply common sense but apparently not that common in our medical system.

If our cells do not receive the nutrients they require to function optimally, then obviously our health and vitality will decline.

For many, this state of semi-starvation manifests in a wide variety of physical and mental symptoms, yet seldom do people consider their symptoms to be partly due to this 1st cause.

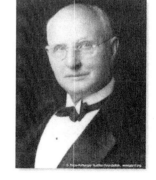

One of the most elegant nutritional research studies was performed by Dr. Weston Price DDS, and supports the first cause of illness stated by Hippocrates.

While practicing dentistry during the late 1800s and early 1900s, Price was curious as to why children presented with far more dental issues than their parents.

15

His practice was during the time of advancing technologies in the processing and manufacturing of foods from companies like Kellogg's and Nabisco.

Price wondered if these dental changes might be due to the introduction and consumption of these less nutritious, industrialized foods.

Therefore, he decided to visit isolated regions of the world, where nutrition was still restricted to locally grown foods.

Dr. Price and his wife traveled to the Swiss Alps, the coast of Scotland, Eskimo and Indian tribes in Canada, the aborigines of Australia, the Maoris of New Zealand, the Amazonian Indians and tribesmen in Africa.

At that time, these indigenous people lived in remote locations far from the influence of 'Western' foods and environmental toxins.

Price kept immaculate and journalistic style notes accompanied by photographs to illustrate his findings.

Price found that in each group, every individual exhibited both dental and physical health.

Infirmities and disease were, for the most part, absent.

Tooth decay was extremely rare and dental crowding was nonexistent.

Over several decades, Price returned to these communities to witness increased dental decay and a variety of chronic illnesses, with the only variable being food stuffs imported by traders and missionaries.

These new foods were primarily white sugar, refined grains, canned foods, pasteurized milk and 'devitalized' fats and oils.

These foods were not only less wholesome and nutritious, but they also displaced the consumption of local foods these people would normally eat.

If you have an interest in learning more about Dr. Price and to understand how our 'modern' foods are at the root of our epidemic in chronic illness, pick up a copy of *Nutrition & Physical Degeneration.*

Environmental Toxins

Hippocrates stated that the 2nd cause of chronic disease was due to our exposure to toxins, and many physicians around the world have confirmed the negative impact environmental chemicals have upon human health.

It seems obvious that when foreign chemicals enter our bodies, in small yet persistent amounts, that over time the body's total burden will increase, and subtle symptoms will become progressively worse.

This is why we must investigate our living, working and surrounding environments, hobbies and gardening activities, food and water sources, mold exposure and even our chronological chemical exposure history.

Just because your symptoms may have developed recently, you must still consider your total accumulation of toxins over your lifetime.

But there are other causes in addition to nutritional deficiencies and environmental toxins which other clinicians since Hippocrates have recognized as causative.

Pathogens

Louis Pasteur ushered in the germ theory, that micro-organisms can be the cause of acute and chronic illnesses.

This is true, but why is it that some people exposed to a virus or bacteria become ill while others do not?

Another 19th century French scientist, Claude Bernard, proposed that it was not just the pathogen but the person's susceptibility to the pathogen which led to illness.

This susceptibility, for why the person's own immune system could not combat the pathogen, relates to a lowered vitality due to the two other causes of illness, nutritional deficiencies and the body's total burden of toxins.

Pathogens (*bacteria, viruses, mold and parasites*) are then the third primary cause of illness.

The problem with assessing this 3rd cause is that, when it comes to a chronic condition, pathogens do not create acute symptoms such as a fever, but rather more benign symptoms such as fatigue.

A person may have had an episode of an acute infection years ago which seemed to clear, but not completely.

Now it's considered a low-grade, silent infection which will fly under the radar and not show up on lab tests.

How to determine if pathogens are an issue will be covered in another section.

Summary

Our medical system has made incredible advances and is certainly necessary at times, yet it is floundering when it comes to treating chronic disease and how to advance a person's health.

Our system creates dependency, seldom asks the patient to take responsibility for their condition, is dogmatic in its opposition to alternative medicine, places a huge financial strain on patients and our nation, negates or neglects the miraculous inner healing capacity of the person and does not address the causes for why a person is ill.

Each person must exercise their common sense and to seek ways of health, ways which will do no harm, and which support their innate physician.

The process of healing and regaining one's full vitality takes time.

Patience, persistence and the practice of a new lifestyle are essential.

For many, illness can become a door through which they discover a calling and an opportunity to see life differently, to become educated and empowered, to pursue a life that resonates more deeply with their heart and soul.

20

NATURE CURE

An ancient principle of medicine is that all true healing comes from nature and that nature provides all the elements the human body requires for health and healing.

Nature provides these elements in the air we breathe, sunlight, the food and herbs we ingest, and the water we drink.

Nature is what we as physicians have called upon for centuries, yet I wish to add an additional perspective.

Yes, nature provides the elements of healing, yet it is the Nature within you, this miraculous wisdom within, which uses and responds to these elements of nature.

The essence of Nature Cure revolves around the body's innate capacity to heal and your role is to assist it by providing what it requires to recover and to preserve your health.

This means becoming more in tune with this wisdom, to listen to its whisperings, to provide what it requires and to avoid what is harmful.

Really, it's that simple.

THE INNATE WISDOM
WITHIN YOU

The Mystery Within

I know this topic was briefly covered before but I believe it bears repeating.

From the moment of your conception this mysterious, innate power ignited the flame of your earthly existence and you, as a 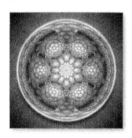 single cell, began to split and multiply into intricate biological and anatomical systems.

Hundreds, then thousands, then millions and trillions of stem cells appeared, taking on a specific function within the hormonal, neurological and skeletal systems, all orchestrated by this mysterious power which has been functioning within you every second of the day and night.

Its intelligence knew exactly how to split one cell into trillions, so without a doubt, it possesses the wisdom to recover your health and to maintain your well-being.

It is your true physician.

To refer to this innate intelligence as a miracle is an understatement for its wisdom can never be truly understood by the finite mind of man.

And what is its essential purpose?

It is to serve you, to help you to live your life with purpose and passion.

But to serve you, it must communicate to you what is beneficial and what is harmful, and you must learn how to listen.

Its language is not through your mother tongue but rather through symptoms, instincts and intuitions.

It also guides you through the whisperings of your conscience.

Deep Into the Core of Chronic Illness

Now we'll dive into the interior of the cell to understand why people experience symptoms due to the three primary causes including pharmaceuticals.

On the physical plane we are composed of over 40 trillion cells and your overall health is a reflection of the sum total function of all these cells.

Therefore, we could say that if your cells are healthy, meaning they are functioning optimally, then you will be symptom free and experiencing health and vitality.

But if their function declines, then symptoms will appear.

Mitochondrial Dysfunction

Inside every cell, except for red blood cells, are small organelles called mitochondria.

These organelles have many functions but the most important is to generate energy (ATP) which drives the cell's function.

If the mitochondria's production of ATP declines, then the function of that cell also declines.

If it's a thyroid cell, then the production of thyroid hormones declines and the person experiences hypothyroid symptoms such as fatigue and depression.

25

If it's a cell that secretes serotonin, then its' production declines and the person may experience depression and insomnia.

As far as recovery and the resurrection of health, the objective must then be to understand the causes of mitochondrial dysfunction and how to correct it.

Causes & Solutions for Mitochondrial Dysfunction

Mitochondria need specific nutrients to function optimally, to make plenty of ATP, and nutritional deficiencies are one cause of lowered mitochondrial function.

These nutrients include most of the B vitamins, various trace minerals and anti-oxidants. Specific foods rich in phytonutrients are essential.

The second cause of mitochondrial dysfunction is the accumulation of toxic residues within the cell, from synthetic chemicals (drugs), many environmental insults, and biotoxins excreted by pathogens.

Even on the cellular level, we must still apply the same holistic principles and methods of recovery and wellness.

AN OVERVIEW OF OUR APPROACH

Now that we've covered some basic principles of health and disease, let's examine some practical steps towards recovery.

In the body there are three compartments of fluid; inside our cells, our lymphatic system and in our blood vessels.

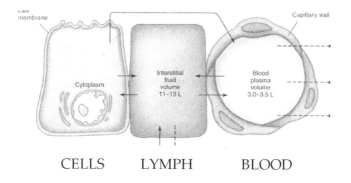

CELLS   LYMPH   BLOOD

On the cellular level, we must use various therapies and nutrition to increase the vitality and function of our cells, which will, in turn, help to excrete toxic residues from within.

The lymph system is also an important part of recovery because when residues are excreted from a cell they will enter the lymph.

It also carries drug and chemical residues into our blood stream to eventually be filtered by our liver and kidneys.

We want our lymph fluid to flow like a river rather than begin stagnant like a swamp.

So how must we take these compartments into account when addressing recovery?

Imagine a very ill woman whose condition is due to a prescription plus the causes we've covered.

- She has a history of eating poorly, of being on a low-caloric, low-fat diet. She has issues with digestion and is likely not assimilating nutrients from her gut. Therefore, all her cells are undernourished and likely under functioning.
- She has been on several prescriptions over the last 5 years and her cells have accumulated toxic residues from these medications and from her environment.
- Her mitochondrial function is less than optimal, and causing some of her symptoms, resulting in poor excretion of drug residues from within her cells.
- Her pathways of detoxification (liver, kidneys, intestines and skin) are compromised and unable to efficiently clear toxins.
- Her lymph system is slow because she is too tired to exercise.
- She has constipation so some toxins filtered from the blood by her liver are likely being reabsorbed back into her body through her intestines.

So where did we start?

Here are the concerns we must consider.

- If we initially use therapies to stimulate her mitochondria in order to help her cells excrete drug residues and accumulated toxins, she would feel much worse because they'll get stuck in her lymph.

- With her lymph being another storage site for toxins, if we use therapies to move her lymph, these toxins will travel into her blood and, again, she will feel worse.
- Toxins filtered by her liver travel to her intestines, and, because she is constipated, many of these toxins will be absorbed back into her body and, again, she'll feel worse.
- So with detoxification (*emptying the bowl*) we need to start downstream from cellular detoxification and, in her case, we must first focus on the colon, one of the primary pathways of detoxification, using various digestive enzymes, probiotics, herbs to improve evacuation, fiber to absorb toxins, and colon hydrotherapy.
- Within a few days we start with lymphatic drainage using massage and hydrotherapy.
- Now we can get to work on removing drug residues and other toxins from her cells. Here we use, among others, a supplement called Mitocore, specifically designed to provide all the nutrients mitochondria require, intravenous NAD, and a few other IVs to improve liver function and to reduce free radicals.
- Throughout this time, we encourage saunas for detoxification through the skin.

Intravenous NAD, or nicotinamide adenine dinucleotide, is a remarkable therapy because of its direct effect on increasing mitochondrial function, but it's important to understand that it should not be a stand-alone therapy for addictions.

I hope I have explained the importance of simultaneously opening the pathways of detoxification, of providing various nutrients and the need for purification therapies, in conjunction with the use of IV NAD.

NAD IV THERAPY: RECOVERING FROM PHARMACEUTICALS

NAD is the most important therapy for recovering from the side-effects of pharmaceuticals and for the restoration of both physical and mental health.

We know these side-effects are due to mitochondrial dysfunction since drug residues and other toxins cause lower energy (ATP) production by the mitochondria, which leads to a decline of cellular function and the inability of the cell to excrete toxic residues.

So, at the very core of recovery, we must increase mitochondrial function

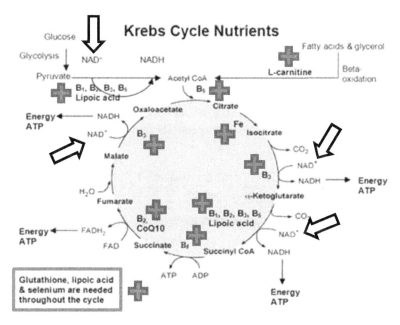

The question then is, 'How do we go about doing this?'

Above is a drawing which illustrates the production of energy within the mitochondria.

Around this clockwise cycle, you'll notice plus signs next to various nutrients which are essential for maximum energy production.

If any of these are deficient then the production of ATP will obviously decline.

Then there are the four broad arrows pointing to NAD.

NAD is the most important step in ATP or energy production.

Remember, the primary goal of recovery is to get chemical and drug residues out of your cells, and their excretion requires an active transport mechanism, meaning that energy (ATP) is required for cellular detoxification.

With NAD, not only are we increasing the vitality of all your cells, but also freeing them from stored toxins.

Various NAD IV Preparations

I was fortunate to spend a couple of days with Dr. Hitt before his passing. His research uncovered the many benefits of using NAD and was the first to use it for recovering from addictions.

There are basically two primary sources or pharmacies that provide NAD for intravenous use.

One source is Anazao Compounding Pharmacy which has the rights to the original Hitt formulas. Unfortunately, these five formulas have been watered down and Anazao will not inform physicians about the concentration of NAD in each of the formulas.

NAD is also known as Coenzyme 1 and other compounding pharmacies are providing this for IV use. We know the exact milligrams of NAD per vial so we can easily adjust the amount of NAD for each client, depending upon their history and present physical and mental condition.

Procedure of Administering NAD

Almost always a person must go through a total of ten consecutive NAD IV sessions.

We always start the 1st IV on a Monday and each day thereafter, skipping Saturday and Sunday after the first week.

In some cases, we will do the Saturday if need be.

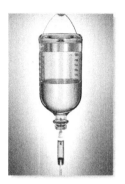

The speed of the IV drip is determined by the degree of discomfort a person experiences in their stomach and small intestines.

The reason for this discomfort is because the cells lining the intestines, where oral pharmaceuticals are absorbed, are the first to react to IV NAD.

These interstitial cells have some of the highest drug residues.

For the first few NAD IVs, many people must throttle the drip rate way down because of abdominal discomfort, and these initial drips may take 6-8 hours.

With each additional IV NAD, the drip rate will be increased, but slow enough so that the IV will not be less than four hours.

Before each NAD IV, we provide a Myers Push, rich in the nutrients mitochondria require.

After each NAD IV, we administer a push of glutathione, an antioxidant.

Since drug residues exiting cells are toxic, glutathione will bind and neutralize them, making it easier for the kidneys and liver to metabolize and process them.

Glutathione is also essential during the two stages of liver detoxification.

Again, NAD is our core therapy for recovering from an addiction to a prescription, and no one will ever recover their optimal health without using this approach.

THE PROCESS OF INVESTIGATION

As one example, I want to walk you through how we approached one case.

As you will see, this case supports the premise that most often, we must first address and correct underlying issues, other than a person's side-effects from their prescription.

A woman in her late 30s was prescribed Citalopram (Celexa), an SSRI, by her physician a year ago for depression.

At that time the physician told her that all her labs were normal, so her condition must be a psychological issue.

For the first six months she had felt somewhat better but then side-effects started to appear;

- Mild weight gain
- A declining interest in sex
- Mild nausea at times
- Her insomnia became worse than before starting the script
- Some drowsiness & fatigue

She had returned to her physician, who wanted to 'try' a different medication but, when she read the possible side-effects, she declined.

She felt trapped but decided to work on her nutrition and to somehow find the energy to exercise. She joined a yoga class and made a greater effort to be with friends.

All the above helped but if she tried weaning off her

35

medication, her symptoms would flare.

When we met she gave many details of her symptoms, which I won't go into.

So, what are the first steps to take with this type of situation?

Do we simply begin he IVs of NAD?

No.

First, we need to know what is going on with her biochemistry and hormones, which means getting some labs.

Here are the highlights.

Thyroid Hormones

Her thyroid hormones (*TSH, T4, Free T4, Free T3 and thyroid antibodies, TPO & TGA*) were within the normal lab range but two of them, one being most important (*Free T3*), was right at the bottom end of the reference range.

A physician would usually interpret these results as normal and pass right over them, but I felt her lower levels were contributing to her fatigue and depression.

I offered her the diagnosis of 'suboptimal hypothyroidism.'

We prescribed a low dose of thyroid medication and a couple of trace minerals to 'feed' her thyroid cells.

Blood Sugar

Besides various nutrients, our cells require two things, oxygen and glucose; no oxygen and we die, no glucose and we slip into a coma.

Could some of her symptoms be due to inadequate glucose or that glucose was not getting into her cells?

A fasting glucose blood test tells us the resting blood sugar after not eating for 12 hours, though it does not tell us what happens to blood sugar after and between meals.

Her fasting glucose result was 72, still within the reference range but not optimal, being 85 to 90.

Another lab test called glycosylated hemoglobin (HA1c) measures the glucose on the hemoglobin protein of red blood cells, and since the life span of a red cell is three months, this result tells us her average blood sugar over the last 90 days.

Her HA1c was 4.5 and if we calculate this to the same units as glucose (*mg/dl*) her average blood glucose was 83.

This meant that, not only is her fasting glucose suboptimal but that she is frequently dipping into low blood sugar or hypoglycemia.

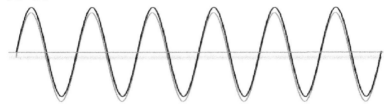

So now we have another cause for her symptoms, that the cells of her body and brain are under functioning because they aren't getting enough glucose when she's in hypoglycemia.

This lady had been concerned with losing weight and had been following a low-caloric, low-fat diet for the last 10 years.

Our nutritionist designed a menu with her, recommending more calories based upon her weight, and increasing her protein and fat intake.

Fats

This brings us to another lab test that might explain why she was experiencing symptoms.

Because of her diet, I suspected a nutrient deficiency that

relates to insomnia, low blood sugar, pain (she had hip pain), fatigue, depression and many others.

All these issues can be due to low levels of two hormones, cortisol and progesterone.

These two hormones, plus a couple of others, are steroid hormones and the glands that make them require a specific nutrient.

What's this vital nutrient these glands require?

Cholesterol.

Low levels of this nutrient will lead to inadequate or suboptimal steroid hormones.

Her lab test for cholesterol was 121 with an optimal being around 185.

Here was another cause for her symptoms.

She had mentioned that her prescribing doctor said her cholesterol was fantastic, that seldom had he seen anyone with this low of a cholesterol result unless they were taking a lipid lowering drug.

'Keep up what you're eating and you'll never die of a heart attack.'

Well, that may be true, but what about quality of life and all the physical and mental symptoms related to low cholesterol and low steroid hormones?

Once this woman understood the necessity of cholesterol, and that it wasn't fats that would make her fat but rather sugars and refined starches, it was an easy shift for her to follow our recommendations.

Vitamin D

Because this woman was very concerned with ageing and

wrinkles, she never went outdoors in the sun for long unless she applied sunscreen.

Her lab result for vitamin D was 28 with an optimal level for a female being 60-70.

Low levels of vitamin D can cause depression, fatigue, and muscle aches and pains.

She was put on 10,000 units a day, of an emulsified form for easy assimilation.

Female Hormones

Upon more detailed questioning, she mentioned that her poor sleep, now and before the prescription, was worse the week before her periods. She also had a greater likelihood of having some minor headaches during this time as well.

We ran saliva hormone testing for one of the estrogens (estradiol) and progesterone.

The results showed a pretty severe progesterone deficiency, maybe due to her low cholesterol, and even though her estradiol was pretty good, she had estrogen dominance, a calculated ratio between her estradiol and progesterone.

The easiest, quickest and most effective way to correct this is to take oral bioidentical progesterone, about 150mgs before bed.

By the way, after just three nights, her sleep had greatly improved.

KPU

Her last unusual lab result was for Kryptopyrroluria or KPU.

Pyrroles are an organic compound which bind Zinc, B6 and other nutrients.

When pyrroles are elevated, this can lead to severe deficiencies of these nutrients.

Zinc acts as an important cofactor in hundreds of biochemical reactions.

B6 is required for neurotransmitter synthesis, especially serotonin, since it is an essential nutrient for mitochondrial function.

A depletion of B6 can lead to various psychological and cognitive issues.

We recommended zinc and both forms of B6, pyridoxine and pyridoxyl-5-phosphate (P5P).

Dark-field Microscope

We viewed a tiny drop of her blood (finger stick) under a dark-field microscope to see if any bacteria, signs of viral issues or mold showed up.

All was clear except for some mold.

We didn't think this was much of an issue compared with the others, yet because she was sensitive to odors and fragrances, we recommended a homeopathic remedy to reduce her sensitivities and to get her home, especially her basement, checked for mold using a test kit from moldcheck.com.

We ran many other labs but the above were the abnormal ones.

We started with supplementation, thyroid hormones, nutritional guidelines, vitamin D, oral progesterone and a few products to improve her liver function and gut ecology.

During the next two weeks we also started her on some

purification therapies including saunas and lymphatic hydrotherapy.

After two weeks she was feeling much better, so we recommended she stop her prescription to begin the 10 days of IV NAD.

She came out of the 10-Day NAD IV Program feeling extremely well.

Comprehensive Lab Testing to Address Underlying Causes

It would be overwhelming, and likely very boring, to list all the labs we run with every client.

So we'll highlight which laboratories we use and some explanation of why.

LabCorp of America

- Lipid Panel for Cholesterol and other fats
- Fasting Glucose
- HA1c
- Liver or Hepatic Panel
- CBC or Complete Blood Count for Red and White Blood Cells
- Comprehensive Metabolic Panel (So many components in this panel)
- Thyroid Hormones
  - TSH
  - T4
  - Free T4
  - Free T3
  - TPO antibodies
  - Thyroglobulin antibodies
  - Reverse T3
- Ferritin for men and post-menopausal women

- C Reactive Protein
- Iron Panel
- Urine analysis
- G6PD (to know if someone can receive high doses of vitamin C intravenously)
- Viral Panel
- Vitamin D
- B12

DHA Laboratory

We run zinc, copper, histamine and the KPU.

The first two, looking for lows and highs, can often relate to psychological issues, with the third to know if someone is an under- or over-methylator.

If they are over or under, then specific supplements are recommended according to the research of Dr. Bill Walsh.

The KPU is to know if the person requires high amounts of specific vitamins and minerals.

Cell Science Systems Lab

Now we are getting down to enzymes related to various pathways of detoxification at the cellular level.

This is a cheek swab for assessing a person's genetic ability or inability to detoxify at the cellular level and whether certain foods or specific nutrients should either be included or excluded.

This panel includes; MTHFR, MTR, MTRR, ACHY and COMT.

Sorry for the abbreviations but their full names would be challenging to pronounce.

Labrix

This lab is used for all our saliva hormone testing.

All hormones in the blood are either attached to a protein carrier, like being on a bus, or they are detached and referred to as free.

Only the free hormones are small enough to leave the blood stream to enter lymph on their way to cells.

In general, and there are a few exceptions, blood lab tests for hormones measure the hormone bound to its protein carrier and the hormone that's free. This is referred to as the total amount of that hormone.

This is true for all the estrogens, progesterone and the adrenal hormone cortisol.

Testing these hormones through blood labs doesn't really tell us how much of the hormone is free and available, which is what we want to know.

Therefore saliva, which is lymph, is the most accurate way to assess certain hormone levels.

Dark-field Microscope

Unless a person has full blown septicemia, which is a severe, systemic bacterial infection, there isn't a blood test that will uncover a low-grade, silent, systemic bacterial infection.

Even the Lyme test has faults, with false negatives (*they actually do have Lyme but the lab results says they don't*) and false positives (*they don't have Lyme but the test says they do*).

We have found the most accurate means of determining if someone has bacteria in their blood is to view a tiny drop of their blood under a dark-field microscope.

Dark-field simply means that when viewing this drop of blood under the microscope, the field, or background, is dark.

This is different from the bright-field microscope used in many hospitals.

When light passes through the microscope's condenser, through the slide and into the lens, any lipid or fat will be illuminated on the viewing monitor.

Bacteria, including spirochetes, have a lipid membrane, so they are easy to spot.

White blood cells are also visible, so we can see their size and activity, helping us to gain some knowledge about the health of a person's immune system.

Mold looks like scum or mucous with white specked highlights, or like a Christmas tree or a fern, also with these white specks.

How we address these pathogens will be covered in another section.

Electrodermal Screening

Dr. Reinhold Voll developed a unit to measure the electrical resistance of acupuncture points.

When a brass stylus or probe is placed directly on a person's acupuncture point, if the corresponding organ or tissue is healthy and vital, then the unit will give a reading of around 50.

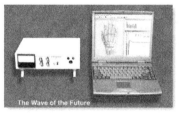

If the reading is above 50, this indicates inflammation or possible infection, usually acute or sub-acute.

Readings less than 50 indicates the corresponding organ or tissue is lower in function and a more chronic condition.

As an example, if there is a low reading on the small intestine acupuncture point it could mean a chronic small intestinal bacterial or fungal overgrowth, a chronic food sensitivity or allergy, leaky gut, or even a parasitic infection.

To determine which it might be, we place various remedies into the circuit while rechecking the point to see which one corrects the low reading.

Therefore, this unit helps to know what the issue is and can also indicate the best approach to treatment.

We use this form of testing to screen for the following;

- Jaw point looking for dental issues
  - Root canals that are infected
  - Heavy metals
  - Cavitations
- Sinus point looking for a chronic sinus infection and whether it's fungal or bacterial
- Tonsil point, checking for a chronic, low-grade infection, even after a tonsillectomy
- Liver for poor detoxification, even when a blood test for liver enzymes is normal
- Small intestines
- Large intestines
- Food allergies

So this covers all the routine testing we do for every person.

Now let's go to all the therapies we offer.

Holistic Therapies To Resolve Underlying Causes

Let's begin this section with an overview of various therapies which address the three primary causes of illness as well as the side-effects from pharmaceuticals.

Nutritional Deficiencies

- IV Vitamins, Minerals & Trace Minerals
- IV Alpha Lipoic Acid
- IV Glutathione Push
- IV BiOcean from France, rich in trace minerals
- IV Meyers Cocktail of Nutrients
- IV Plaquex for Cellular Membrane Repair

Environmental Toxins, Drug Residues & Biotoxins

Cellular Detoxification

- IV NAD
- IV Glutathione Push

General Detoxification (Emptying the Bowl)

- IV Alpha Lipoic Acid
- Lymphatic Hydrotherapy
- The Bemer for Clearing Lymph and the Matrix
- Colon Hydrotherapy
- Walk-in Sauna with Cold Shower

Pathogens (bacteria, spirochetes, viruses & mold)

- IV Zotzmann 10-Pass Ozone Therapy
- IV UBI (Ultraviolet Blood Photonic Therapy)
- IV UVLRx (Direct Venous Ultraviolet Therapy)
- IV High Dose Vitamin C

Let's cover, in more detail, each of the above IV therapies.

Nutritional IVs

The Multivitamin, Mineral & Trace Mineral IV provides all
the B-vitamins, various minerals like
magnesium, calcium and potassium, and
trace minerals such as zinc, manganese and
selenium.

Alpha Lipoic Acid improves mitochondrial
activity and specifically helps to repair liver
cells, and to improve their function. Lipoic
acid is also an antioxidant and can potentiate
the benefits of the IV vitamin C when administered
afterwards.

Glutathione is an antioxidant and helps neutralize free
radicals and improve the liver's ability to clear toxins from the
blood. It is given as a push from a syringe directly into the
vein.

BiOcean from France is deep ocean water,
harvested and then processed through a
sophisticated cold-filtration system leaving all
minerals and trace minerals intact.

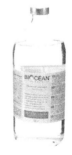

Meyers Cocktail is a quick and simple means
of delivering vitamin C, various minerals and

B vitamins intravenously.

It is also referred to as a Meyers Push since these ingredients are drawn into a 60cc syringe rather than a large IV bag. The speed of delivery is slow and takes about 10 minutes.

Plaquex has been used for over 55 years in about one-quarter of the world's countries and was originally developed to resolve fatty embolus (plaque) during and after surgery.

In the 1990s its use shifted to complement IV EDTA chelation therapy, used for removing or dissolving hardened plaque from the walls of arteries.

Not only does Plaquex help repair the lining of arteries, it also improves the membranes surrounding all our cells.

A healthier cell membrane allows increased waste excretion and the uptake of vital nutrients.

Plaquex is designed to repair cell membranes that have been damaged by toxic substances, drugs, heavy metals, solvents and free radicals.

IVs for Environmental & Drug Toxins

NAD IVs are the primary means of getting drug residues and other toxins to be excreted from inside every cell of the body and brain.

This topic was already covered in a previous section.

IVs for Pathogens

To discover if a person has issues with blood pathogens we use both standard lab testing and looking at a tiny drop of a client's blood sandwiched between two pieces of glass (a microscope slide and a cover slip) under a dark-field microscope.

To address bacteria, including spirochetes, viruses and mold, we use the following IV therapies.

Zotzmann 10-Pass Hyperbaric Ozone Therapy

This treatment mimics the activity of our own white blood cells.

To kill pathogens, our white blood cells produce hydrogen peroxide, which is H_2O_2.

This molecule breaks down into H_2O (water) and a singlet oxygen. This single oxygen atom is what kills or oxidizes pathogens.

Ozone is O_3 and breaks down into O_2 and the same singlet oxygen.

Ozone and H_2O_2 reduce not only bacteria but mold as well, and cripple viruses to inhibit their replication.

Ozone has other health benefits including the increased oxygen carrying capacity of red blood cells and improving the function of mitochondria.

The German Zotzmann machine allows us to treat about 2,000cc of a client's blood with ozone during a single session, which takes between one to two hours.

After almost two years of experimenting and comparing a client's blood before and after the Zotzmann using the dark-field microscope, we find the best results are when the Zotzmann 10-pass is followed by a high dose IV vitamin C, around 6 to 16 hours after the Zotzmann.

UBI or Bio-Photonic Therapy

This treatment uses ultraviolet light to treat about 100cc of blood.

This therapy has been in use by physicians for over 70 years.

There have been over a million treatments given and not a single adverse reaction recorded.

Some proven benefits of this therapy are the following:

- Kills bacteria and molds in the blood
- Inhibits the replication of viruses
- Supercharges the immune system
- Improves microcirculation
- Oxygenates tissues
- Reduces inflammation
- Stimulates red blood cell production
- Increases the flexibility of red blood cells and therefore better oxygen delivery to tissues

We extract 100cc of blood from a client's vein into a sterile, disposable syringe. This blood is then transferred into a sterile IV bag filled with 120cc of sterile 0.9% sodium chloride.

We then inject 100cc of ozone into this blood/sodium chloride mixture.

This final mix flows from the IV bag through a sterile IV line attached to a special 12" Turbo 180 cuvette which is inserted into our GHL 3000 ultraviolet unit, and back into the vein.

At no time is the catheter or needle removed from the client's vein, so every step remains sterile.

UVLRx

This IV therapy is similar to the UBI therapy; to reduce pathogens, viruses and mold.

Instead of extracting blood from the vein, as with the UBI, the UVLRx delivers specific UV frequencies directly to the blood through a thin, sterile, single-use fiber optic inserted through a soft catheter already placed in the vein.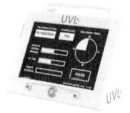

To keep the tip of this fiber optic clear of platelet aggregation, we must simultaneously provide an IV drip of sterile 0.9% sodium chloride which flows across this tip.

We found that if we ozonate this sodium chloride and simultaneously drip this sterile ozonated fluid during the UVLRx, then the outcome is even better.

During the one-hour treatment, almost all the blood in the body is being treated by these UV frequencies.

The UVLRx is computer driven to deliver three very specific frequencies.

Whether to use the Zotzmann, the UBI or the UVLRx will depend upon the individual, the results of the dark-field microscope and the size of the client's vein.

High-Dose Vitamin C

This IV delivers upwards of 25 grams of C, over an hour and a half.

Vitamin C in high doses, delivered intravenously, is an oxidative therapy.

Therefore, this administration acts similar to the other oxidative therapies mentioned above.

For the best results of reducing pathogens, we combine high-dose vitamin C with the Zotzmann, UBI and the UVLRx, as long as there is a period of time between them, anywhere from 6 to 18 hours.

There is another reason why we administer vitamin C after these other therapies.

Ozone and UV light kill off a lot of pathogens which are then circulating throughout the blood stream. These dead pathogens must be cleared or cleaned up by our white blood cells.

Vitamin C nourishes and stimulates our white blood cells to consume these dead pathogens, a process called phagocytosis.

This covers all the intravenous therapies and the reasons for their use.

Now, let's review other therapies for purification and recovery.

PURIFICATION THERAPIES FOR RECOVERY

This chapter covers therapies which assist detoxification pathways to rid the body of drug and chemical residues.

To refresh your memory, toxins are located in various tissues.

- Inside every cell of the body and brain.
- Fat cells just under the skin are another storage site.
- Residues are found in the cells lining of the small intestines, called the Enteric Nervous System.
- Lymph fluid is another site of chemical and drug residues.

As mentioned earlier, before we begin to mobilize drug residues from inside our cells, it's important to move or drive the lymph system (clear the swamp).

Lymphatic Hydrotherapy

An old time naturopathic therapy with multiple benefits is the application of hot and cold compresses to the upper body, first introduced by two naturopathic physicians, Dr. Carroll and Dr. Harold Dick.

I was very fortunate to do part of my clinical internship with Dr. Dick.

When I arrived, I thought I'd just be an observer and pick up some clinical pearls along the way.

But he told me if I really wanted to understand the benefits of hydrotherapy, I'd have to experience it.

So twice a day, for three days, I also became his patient.

I tell you… after three days I felt amazing and I decided to continue the therapy with the help of another student for seven more days after returning to school.

I will walk through each step of the treatment to explain its benefits and why it is the best therapy to move lymph fluid and to drain the swamp.

The Procedure

You lie on your back on a massage table, undressed from the waist up, and covered with wool blankets from your neck to your feet.

The hydrotherapist uncovers your chest and abdomen, and places a moist hot compress from just below the neck to the pubic bone.

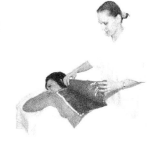

The blankets are adjusted to cover the hot compress and tucked tightly around the sides of the neck, shoulders, chest and waist.

This heating compress remains for five minutes.

What is the body's response to this hot compress?

When heat is applied to the skin it causes a reddening, since fresh blood circulates into the small capillary blood vessels just under the skin.

But something else is going on here.

Over the entire body we have dermatomes which run in parallel lines along our skin. These dermatomes are rich in nerves which reflect, through the spinal column, deep into the body.

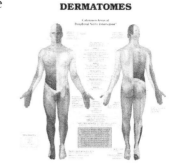

DERMATOMES

When a dermatome on the skin is heated, its corresponding internal organ(s), reacts in a similar way, with increased blood flow.

Heat placed on the skin, say at dermatomes 7, 8 and 9, will cause the dilation of blood vessels within the liver, with the corresponding increase in blood flow.

With the application of a hot compress over the chest and abdomen, all the underlying organs will be filled with fresh blood causing increased oxygenation, increased delivery of nutrients and the removal of metabolic waste and toxins.

After five minutes, the hot compress is replaced by a cold compress, covering the same area of the chest and abdomen.

This cold compress remains for 10 minutes.

Now what is happening?

The body's <u>initial</u> reaction to a cold compress is the opposite of the heating compress.

The blood vessels just under the skin constrict, driving blood into the core of the body.

This same reaction is occurring to the internal organs as well since the dermatomes are sending a chilling or constricting message.

This is the initial, immediate reaction to cold (constriction) but then there's a <u>secondary</u> reaction.

The body will, after a few minutes, redirect blood to the skin to warm the cold compress.

As fresh warm blood is flowing to the skin, the same is happening to the internal organs.

This pumping action, of blood flowing back and forth to the skin and in and out of the organs, has many benefits including purification.

This alternating of hot and cold also increases the activity of what's called the 'lymphatic pump.'

To activate this pump even further, we use a sine wave machine which causes a gentle contraction and relaxation of the muscles along the spine and over the center section of the abdomen.

After the hot and cold compresses to the chest and abdomen, you then turn onto your front and the same procedure, the 5-minute hot compress followed by the 10-minute cold compress, is repeated.

This therapy not only increases the flow of lymph but also improves digestive issues, blood sugar dysregulation and liver, gall bladder and kidney drainage.

Colon Hydrotherapy

The intestinal tract is one of the primary routes the body uses to expel drug residues and toxins, and must therefore be considered during purification.

When toxins are metabolized and filtered from the blood by the liver, they first pass through the gall bladder on their way to the small intestines.

Once these toxins reach the gut they must then travel the entire length of the intestines, which is about 20 feet.

The faster we can move these toxins through the gut the less likely they will be absorbed back into the body.

During a purification program, as toxins are being released from cells, and the lymph is dumping them into the blood stream, a person can feel unwell.

With colon hydrotherapy we can immediately reduce unpleasant detoxification symptoms.

The Procedure

We use a three-stage water filtration system.

The water is kept at body temperature and flows, at a very low pressure, through a sterile disposable speculum inserted into the rectum.

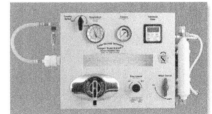

This is a closed system so there is no odor at all.

As the water slowly fills the colon, it works its way up the left side and then across the transverse colon.

At some point the person feels the urge to evacuate.

The therapist opens a valve on the unit to allow all the fluid and fecal material from the colon to flow out the tubing and through an illuminated transparent glass tube in the machine.

This viewing may reveal undigested food, oil or fat globules, signs of Candida, and parasites.

Our colon hydrotherapists are fully trained and certified, with years of experience.

Saunas to the Rescue

I sincerely believe that if saunas were incorporated into our modern lifestyle, we would not be witnessing such a rapid decline in the health of our population.

Even the issues of pharmaceutical side-effects could be greatly improved since a lot of their residues are compartmentalized within fat cells just under our skin.

Getting drug and chemical residues out of this layer is easily accomplished through perspiration.

But a word of caution.

If heat penetrates too deeply, then some toxins released from fat cells will enter the body rather than out through the skin.

For this reason, we prefer the dry heat sauna over the infrared.

The Benefits of Sauna

For centuries saunas have been used by various cultures for purification, relaxation, spiritual rites and connecting with nature.

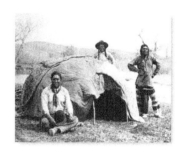

Yet how often do we sweat?

We go from our air-conditioned homes to our air-conditioned cars.

Many of us do not have a job that requires physical exertion and therefore we do not sweat.

We use antiperspirants and apply skin creams which leave residues that block the pores of our sweat glands.

So, saunas, if we are to improve our health, must become a part of our lifestyle.

The Sauna Experience

During the sauna experience you should feel completely relaxed. Therefore, perspiring during exercise will not be as beneficial compared with relaxing in a sauna.

We want blood to flow to our skin and not necessarily to our muscles.

This is key.

The more relaxed our muscles are the easier blood will flow from the body's core to the skin's surface.

This easier flow keeps the heart calm and maintains a lower heart rate and blood pressure.

Walk-in Dry Sauna

Our walk-in sauna is private unless you request another to join you.

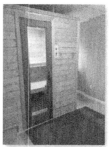

There is plenty of room to lie down and to relax.

Next to our walk-in sauna is a shower.

If you remember the benefits of the alternating hot and cold compresses with Lymphatic Hydrotherapy, you will understand why we have located the shower so close to the sauna.

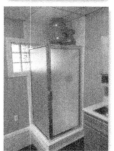

It's best to alternate between the hot sauna and a cold shower.

After working up a good sweat, and you sense the body would like a refreshing cool rinse, you exit the sauna and enter the shower.

This cold stimulates your mitochondria and the release of stem cells.

This cold rinse also prepares you for additional time in the sauna.

We recommend going back and forth between the sauna and the cold shower, always starting with the sauna and finishing with cold, and doing three cycles; hot/cold, hot/cold, and hot/cold.

The last cold can be warmer since it's important to remove oils from the skin using a chemical free soap.

Our Sauna Detox Program

To accentuate the benefits of the sauna detox, we recommend taking vitamin B3 (niacin) and an oral supplement to bind any toxins in the gut.

Vitamin B3 causes a flushing of the skin, especially the upper part of the body. This flushing means increased circulation and the delivery of oxygen to cells.

B3 is also an important cofactor in the production of ATP.

The Bemer

Dr. Alfred Pischinger, MD (1899-1982) from Austria was the first scientist to describe the regulation of the Extracellular Matrix (ECM) and stated that health and disease are determined by the state or quality of this Matrix tissue which includes the lymph system, or lymph fluid, and the fluid in the capillaries.

If this Matrix is clean and free of toxins, then the person will most likely remain healthy.

If it is unclean then the person will most likely become ill.

If the Matrix is running like a stream, then drug residues and toxins excreted by cells will more easily be swept away.

Besides Lymphatic Hydrotherapy, what else can we do?

Let's talk about the capillaries, our smallest blood vessels, which are part of this Matrix.

As arteries become smaller (arterioles) and smaller we finally come to the tiny capillaries through which red blood cells flow to deliver oxygen and to carry away waste.

Before each capillary is a tiny muscle called the pre-capillary sphincter.

If this muscle is tight then red cells and blood flow are restricted.

What if we could help this tiny, pre-capillary muscle to relax?

Its relaxation would allow more red blood cells to flow through, thus delivering more oxygen to increase mitochondrial function and an increased clearing of toxic residues.

A German company was given the task of improving the health of the older population to reduce government spending on health care.

They developed the Bemer, which emits, what they call, micro-Tesla frequencies to specifically relax this pre-capillary sphincter or muscle.

A Bemer treatment lasts eight-minutes, where a person lies on a full-length mat which emits these frequencies.

Besides the benefits mentioned, we use the Bemer before each IV therapy to enhance the delivery of nutrients to tissues.

THE PSYCHOLOGY OF RECOVERY

By Dr. Haskell's daughter, Justyn Manley, LCSW

You may be asking, "How do we incorporate the psychological component of recovery?"

You may be thinking, "I've tried therapy before, but it didn't seem to work," or "What's the point of sitting around and talking about all the things that have happened in the past, are happening now, or what might happen in the future?"

As a psychotherapist, I have heard these words time and time again when first meeting a client.

I am therefore writing this chapter from the perspective of a human being and a psychotherapist, to express the reasons I think therapy is important, and what my experiences have been as a person providing this specific service to fellow human beings.

In my practice I like to use metaphors.

Let's start with one that might aid in understanding therapy.

Let's say there is a suit of armor, which represents your painful experiences, and at some point you decide, metaphorically, to put that suit of armor in the closet.

You avoid taking it out, because thinking and feeling about it is too painful to deal with it, and it's left in the closet for a long time.

Over time that suit of armor, or those painful experiences, not only gathers dust, but it tarnishes and corrodes. Sometimes the armor in the closet may come to mind and it evokes anxiety or depression.

But trying to push it away fuels the anxiety or depression, which means the anxiety or depression is growing in intensity as we push painful experiences and memories away.

Then we do all sorts of things to deal with that growing intensity, like working constantly, using drugs or alcohol, over or under eating, exercising to extremes, trying to control others, and many other ways of avoidance.

These attempts will often work in the short term, to feel some relief, but that suit of armor in the closet is still there.

During this process, all the ways we try to avoid thinking and feeling about that suit of armor, moves us further and further away from the things that matter most to us.

The reason I tell this story and describe it metaphorically, is that therapy is about taking that suit of armor out of the closet, holding it, touching it, being with it, and polishing off the tarnish and corrosion.

A client and therapist will work together, to purposefully find ways to feel, think, and approach those painful experiences.

It can be terrifying and very difficult work, but without a purposeful approach, there is often a strong distraction from the life a person wants to be living.

I want to say something about two important aspects of the purposeful work that is done.

Together, the past experiences, which likely link to an addiction, are brought out of that dark closet and into the light. By being with the past, it loses much of its power, with less desire to avoid it in unhealthy ways, with it becoming no longer the monster in the closet.

Once the hard work is done, when a memory comes to mind,

the tendency will no longer be to avoid it. The feelings of fear or guilt or anger that were once associated with those painful experiences, no longer have the same power.

Let's talk about the 'purposeful approach' part of therapy and how it actually works.

As an example, let's address all the physical and mental sensations that come up when we desire to take a prescription or a drug.

These sensations are triggered by molecules and hormones circulating in your blood that travels throughout your body and brain. These sensations are somewhat pleasurable and yet you wish they would disappear.

You try to ignore them because you want to change your life and to be free, and to stop hiding and lying.

And then there's the guilt.

You know your life and your relationships with loved ones would improve if only you could be free.

You might try to distract yourself, to keep on the move, but that nagging feeling of desire just gets stronger.

The purposeful approach begins with developing mindfulness, the ability to observe, without judgement, the feelings associated with addiction, including desire, guilt, discontent, self-criticism and a sense of being out of control.

This sense of detachment from these sensations is mixed with curiosity and hope.

Together, we find an appropriate metaphor and use various treatment options which aid in reprocessing, organizing, and approaching this addiction.

Treatment also includes awareness around to how the addiction has impacted your beliefs about yourself, others and the world.

We also identify what beliefs are now getting in the way of living a higher quality of life.

We address past events by approaching future real life situations.

Wearing my human being hat, when I sit with a client and we explore together, this is where the work I do is deeply meaningful. It is with great gratitude that I do this work and to have others trust me enough to join them on their journey.

When we are in the room, there is this mutual sense of being very grounded in that moment, that feels important and notable to express.

What I have discovered after many years of providing psychotherapy, one human being to another, is that people are so relieved to do this in a purposeful, mindful way.

Once the perceived threat of feeling, thinking and talking about their addiction is resolved, there is a palpable shift in the person which can be felt in the room. Experiencing that with someone is why I do this work.

You may be asking how a psychotherapist does this works year after year and I say, as people address their desires and emotions, approach them and reprocess them, I also experience resolve alongside that person.

It is my hope that sharing these thoughts sparks curiosity about how psychotherapy could be helpful for you.

Justyn's specialty training includes EMDR (Eye Movement Desensitization and Reprocessing), Cognitive Processing Therapy, Prolonged Exposure, and Cognitive-Behavioral Conjoint Therapy, which are all treatments for PTSD.

SUMMARY & HIGHLIGHTS

Here are some highlights of what's been covered.

- The symptoms you associate with your prescription are due to many causes and not just the medication.
- Most conditions are due to nutritional deficiencies, harmful environmental toxins including pharmaceuticals, and pathogens.
- These three causes lead to mitochondrial dysfunction.
- The primary way to decrease physical and mental symptoms is to eliminate drug and toxic residues from inside your cells.
- Reduce your exposure to chemicals and environmental toxins.
- Use various purification therapies to help your body to excrete toxins.
- Use intravenous therapies to improve nutrient levels, to support the immune system, to reduce pathogens and environmental toxins, and to improve the pathways of detoxification.
- Remember, you possess a miraculous innate physician which is dedicated to helping you to recover your health.
- Secure a mental attitude of respect and appreciation for this wisdom.
- This wisdom speaks to you through physical and mental symptoms, your conscience, intuition, instincts and common sense.

- It is your responsibility to support this wisdom and to learn its language.
- Realize that the vitality deep within your body and soul can never be restored through artificial means.
- Invest in your health otherwise your savings and income will be consumed by medical expenses.

How to Become a Client

If you are interested in coming to our clinic, to take advantage of our services and therapies, this is how to proceed.

If you live close to our clinic then read the first section.

If you are from out of state, there are several things which must be done before your arrival. Go to the next section titled 'Long-Distance Clients'.

Clients in Utah

When you call our clinic and mention your interest in our program for treating side-effects from pharmaceuticals, our receptionist will forward our intake questionnaire to your email address.

Complete this questionnaire on your computer, save it and attach it to an email to us at AdvancingCare@gmail.com.

Dr. Haskell will review your answers and will then contact you by phone to cover any questions you might have.

An appointment will be scheduled for a blood draw along with instructions regarding preparation.

You will also be asked to bring a urine sample.

When you come for the blood draw, you will also receive additional kits for collecting specimens at home.

- Saliva kit for various hormones
- Urine kit for checking KPU

- Cheek swab kit, checking for MTHFR (*both heterozygous & homozygous*), MTR (*both heterozygous & homozygous*), MTRR (*heterozygous*), AHCY (*homozygous*) and COMT.

When all results have arrived, your first clinic appointment will be scheduled with Dr. Haskell, his assistant, our nutritionist and his daughter, Justyn Manley.

During this two-hour consultation with Dr. Haskell, the following will be covered;

- A detailed review of your symptoms
- A review and explanation of lab results, what they mean and ways to correct them
- Viewing a drop of your blood under a dark-field microscope
- Testing various acupuncture points on our EAV unit.
- Likely a brief physical exam
- Recommendations for various supplements or products to address underlying issues reflected in the lab reports and to improve your pathways of detoxification
- Prioritization of the most important therapies to begin with will also be clarified
- Determining when you will be ready to start the ten days of IV NAD.

Dr. Haskell might suggest a number of nutritional IVs, and possibly to begin addressing blood pathogens or mold with the 10-pass Zotzmann, UBI or UVLRx.

You will come away with a very clear agenda, a timeline of how you will proceed along the path to recovery.

Each person is different in terms of how long it takes to do the entire program including the 10 NAD IVs at the end.

Figure that from the time of your 1st consult to completing the

10 NAD IVs will be around a month.

Everything is included in this program up to and including the last IV NAD.

- Dr. Haskell's review of your intake questionnaire.
- All blood, urine, saliva and cheek swab genetic testing
- The initial two-hour consultation with Dr. Haskell
- The one-hour visit with our nutritionist.
- The initial one-hour consult with Justyn Manley plus four additional visits
- A half-hour consultation mid-way through the program with Dr. Haskell
- A repeat of the dark-field microscope if progress needs to be assessed
- All supplements during the program, up until the last NAD IV
- All IVs which address the three primary causes of illness.
- All nutritional IVs already covered
- IVs to reduce pathogens (Zotzmann, UBI and UVLRx)
- Ten NAD IVs
- All purification therapies
  - Colon hydrotherapy
  - Lymphatic hydrotherapy
  - The Bemer
  - Saunas

At the time of this writing, the cost of the complete program is $10,000USD.

Long Distance Clients

When you call our clinic and mention your interest in our program for treating side-effects from pharmaceuticals, our receptionist will forward our intake questionnaire to your email address.

Complete this questionnaire on your computer, save it and attach it to an email to us at AdvancingCare@gmail.com.

Dr. Haskell will review your answers to the questionnaire and call you to cover any questions you might have.

His assistant will then reach out to you to explain your next steps which involve lab testing.

We will then forward a LabCorp of America requisition with instructions on how to locate one of their patient service centers and how to prepare for the blood draw.

We will also forward additional kits by mail for collecting specimens at home.

- Saliva kit for various hormones
- Urine kit for checking KPU
- Cheek swab, checking for MTHFR (*both heterozygous & homozygous*), MTR (*both heterozygous & homozygous*), MTRR (*heterozygous*), AHCY (*homozygous*) and COMT.

When all lab results arrive to us, they will be forwarded to you as attachments to your email address.

We will then contact you to schedule your first one-hour consultation with Dr. Haskell and his assistant.

These will be long-distance appointments because we want you to get started with our program before you arrive, to be sure you will receive the most benefits from all our therapies including the IV NAD.

During this consultation, the following will be covered.

- A detailed review of your symptoms
- A review and explanation of your lab results, what they mean and ways correct them.
- Recommendations for various supplements or products to start before you arrive which address some underlying issues reflected in your lab reports
- Products will also be suggested to begin improving your pathways of detoxification.
- Advice about some therapies you might start before your arrival
- Determining when you will be ready to come to the clinic to begin all our therapies including the IVs of NAD.

You will come away from this initial long-distance consult with a very clear agenda, the steps you'll take along the path to recovery.

Your long-distance consult with our nutritionist will be coordinated with Dr. Haskell and his findings from labs and his consult with you.

Your initial consult with Justyn Manley will also be long-distance. This will likely be a brief conversation, with the other's scheduled when you arrive.

When you arrive at our clinic, you will have another visit with Dr. Haskell to review how you are doing, to view a drop of your blood under the dark-field microscope, a brief physical exam and testing a few acupuncture points.

An agenda for therapies will be discussed and scheduled.

You will need to be with us for a minimum of two weeks since the IV NAD requires 10 sessions, Monday through Friday and then the following Monday through Friday.

But ideally a long-distance person would come for three weeks because we might find issues with blood pathogens and mold which would require several ozone, UBI or UVLRx treatments.

Trying to schedule these IVs as well as the ten NAD IVs is really challenging for both you and our staff if you are here for only two weeks.

Everything is included in our program up to and including the last IV NAD.

- Dr. Haskell's review of your intake questionnaire
- All blood, urine, saliva and genetic cheek swab testing
- The initial long-distance hour consultation with Dr. Haskell over the phone
- A one-hour consultation with Dr. Haskell when you arrive, which includes the dark-field microscope and EAV testing
- A repeat of the dark-field microscope if we need to assess progress
- One hour consult with our nutritionist
- One hour consult with Justyn Manley and four others while you are here
- All supplements shipped to you long-distance as well as any supplements Dr. Haskell recommends after seeing you in our clinic, up until the last NAD IV
- All IVs
  - All those listed in this book
  - IVs to reduce pathogens (Zotzmann, UBI and UVLRx)
  - Ten NAD IVs

- All purification therapies
  - Colon hydrotherapy
  - Lymphatic hydrotherapy
  - The Bemer
  - Saunas

At the time of this writing, the cost of the complete program is $10,000USD, whether you come for two or three weeks to our clinic.

We are an out-patient facility, but you will be sent our 'Hospitality Welcome Package' listing lodging, restaurants, entertainment and local, nature destinations.

Please feel free to reach out to us if you have any questions.

Printed in Great Britain
by Amazon

57126933R00050